The Purpose of this Book.

When the electrical system of the heart fails to work properly, we can assist the heart by implanting electrical leads into regions of the heart to provide the necessary electrical stimulus for muscle contraction.

These electrical stimuli must go through the muscle itself and as such the pattern displayed on the electrocardiogram resembles that seen with bundle branch block morphology. You will notice that the conventionally placed ventricular lead is in the right ventricle.

This means – as you should remember from the prior books on reading electrocardiograms – the morphology will appear as a left bundle as the electrical stimulus will begin in the right ventricle and then travel through the walls of the left ventricle.

Initially these electrical leads were powered by external sources and vacuum tubes (aka the Fleming valve) invented by Professor John Ambrose Fleming in 1904.

Today these leads are powered by implantable sources that are closely monitored and replaced every 3-7 years depending upon what is required from the battery sources.

In this brief tutorial we will look at the nomenclature of pacemakers and what is seen on the electrocardiogram.

I dedicate this book to my friend and teacher, Dr. Denton Arthur Cooley with whom I had the privilege of sharing patient care.

Basic Pacemakers

By: Dr. Richard M. Fleming
Physicist – Nuclear Cardiologist

Temporary vs. Permanent

- **Temporary**
  - Covers emergency or temporary situations
    - Eg. idioventricular rhythm associated with MI
    - Eg. bridge the gap while drugs are wearing off
  - Types
    - External
    - Internal
      - Usually Internal Jugular (Right)
- **Permanent**
  - Placed under fluoroscopy, frequently left subclavian
  - May include AICD

Basic Nomenclature

- Threshold
  - The minimal energy necessary to produce the desired effect (viz. production of electrical current in the heart). AKA "capture"
- Output
  - The energy output set to guarantee threshold
    - 2-3 x the threshold level
- Sensitivity
  - The ability of the pacemaker to detect the intrinsic activity of the heart.

Basic Nomenclature (cont):

- Rate
  - The rate at which one sets the pacer to activate if the heart does not.
- Delay
  - The amount of time the pacemaker is told to wait before doing something.
    - Eg. How long to wait after a P-wave before activating an electrical stimulus for the ventricles.
      - Eg. would you wait 80 mSec, 120 mSec, 200 mSec, 300 mSce.

Basic Nomenclature (cont):

- The more you ask the computer to do, the more battery power you will use, the sooner the battery will fail and it will need to be replaced.
- EOL = End of life
  - Of the battery, hopefully not the patient.
  - When this happens, the pacer rate slows down & then default to a non-sensing fixed-pacing mode.

Failures

- Battery failure, lead displacement, lead fracture, a magnet is placed over the computer.
- Failure to sense
  - The native electrical activity of the heart is not detected by the pacemaker
  - Due to low p-wave amplitude
  - Fibrosis after the lead is implanted
  - Fracture of pacemaker wire/lead insulation
- Treatment
  - Correcting damaged wire
  - Increasing sensitivity, although, this may result in oversensing and inappropriate pauses

Failures (cont):

- Oversensing
  - Failure to initiate an electrical pacer response when needed.
    - Iatrogenic (we've set it too sensitive and it sees everything as cardiac electrical activity)
    - Shows up as absence of pacemaker spikes
  - Usually resulting from
    - Lead fracture (no information coming from the pacer computer)
    - Sensing of myopotentials of skeletal muscle
    - Cross-talk (ventricular lead interprets atrial pacer activity as ventricular activity)

Failures (cont):

- Failure to capture
  - The pacemaker fires and there is no resultant electrical stimulation of the heart.
  - Caused by:
    - Lead migration
    - Rise in threshold (scarring around pacer lead)
  - Rx
    - Correcting underlying cause
    - Temporarily increasing output

Failures (final):

- Pacemaker mediated tachycardia (PMT).
    - Dual chamber pacemakers
    - The atrial lead senses a retrograde p-wave and initiates a pacing cycle, which causes another retrograde p-wave and the cycle (tachycardia) continues.
    - Rx
        - Change to VVI.
- Pacemaker syndrome
    - VVI pacemaker results in fixed rate and with dysynergy between atrial and ventricles, the atrial contract against closed valves and further compromise in cardiac output.

The Magic Five-Letter Code

- The first letter – Chambers paced.
  - Where the activity will come from
  - A=atrium, V=ventricle, D=both
- The second letter – Chambers sensed.
  - Where the pacemaker is looking for native activity
  - A=atrium, V=ventricle, D=both

The Magic Five-Letter Code (cont):

- The third letter – Mode of response to chambers sensed
  - I=inhibited (don't fire, we're going fast enough)
  - T=triggered (fire when not going fast enough)
  - D=dual (does both)

The Magic Five-Letter Code (cont):

- The fourth letter – Programmability
  - P=programmed rate or output only.
  - M=multi-programmable
    - Multiple information/instructions
  - 0=no programming (dummy system)
- The fifth letter – response to tachycardia
  - R=rate response
    - Slowly increases rate as needed to keep up with physiologic needs
  - B=burst
    - Rapid increase in heart rate

Examples of Pacemakers

- VVI
  - Intermittent backup for inactive patient
  - Advantages
    - Cheap, simple
  - Disadvantages
    - Fixed rate, potential pacemaker syndrome

Examples of Pacemakers

- VVIR
  - Useful for atrial fibrillation
  - Advantages
    - Rate responsiveness
  - Disadvantages
    - Requires appropriate programming

Examples of Pacemakers

- DDD
  - Useful for complete heart block
  - Advantage
    - Atrial tracking restores normal physiology
  - Disadvantage
    - If brady-tachy syndrome, no rate responsivenes
    - Requires two leads
    - More programming

Examples of Pacemakers

- DDDR
  - Useful for need for rate responsiveness
    - Eg. AV block
  - Advantages
    - All options available
  - Disadvantages
    - Complex programming

Atrial Pacing

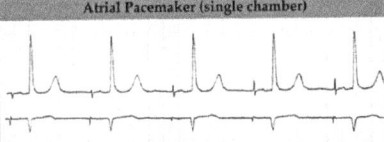

Atrial Pacemaker (single chamber)

One spike producing an abnormal P wave (atrial capture) followed by a normal QRS

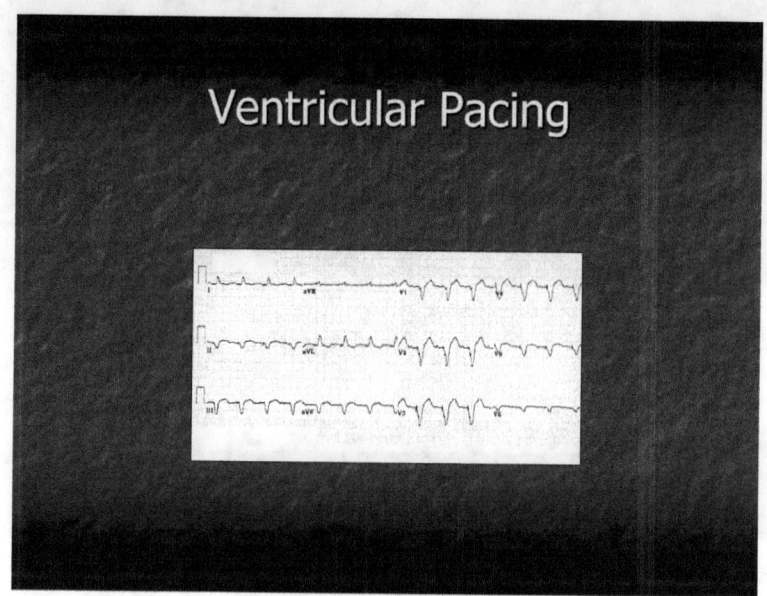

AV Sequential Pacing

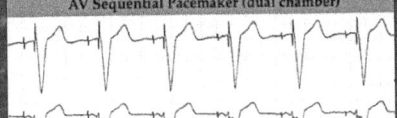

One spike followed by an abnormal P (atrial capture) followed by a Second spike producing a wide QRS (ventricular capture).

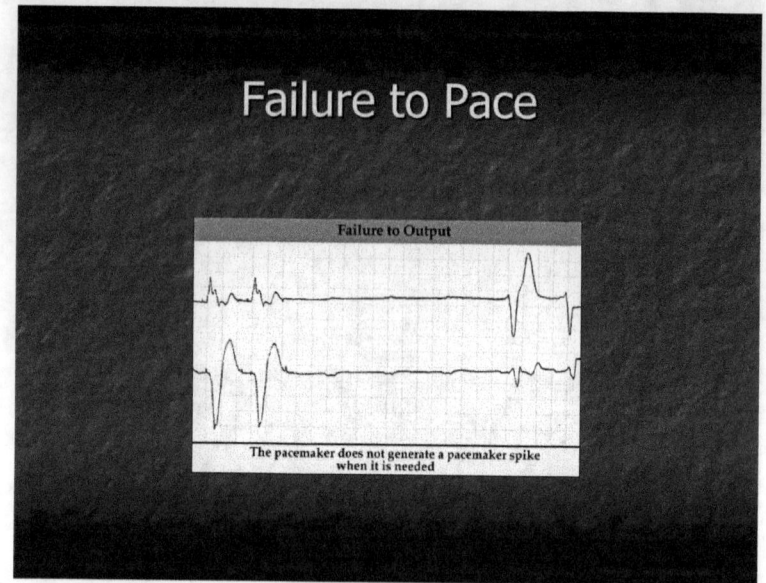

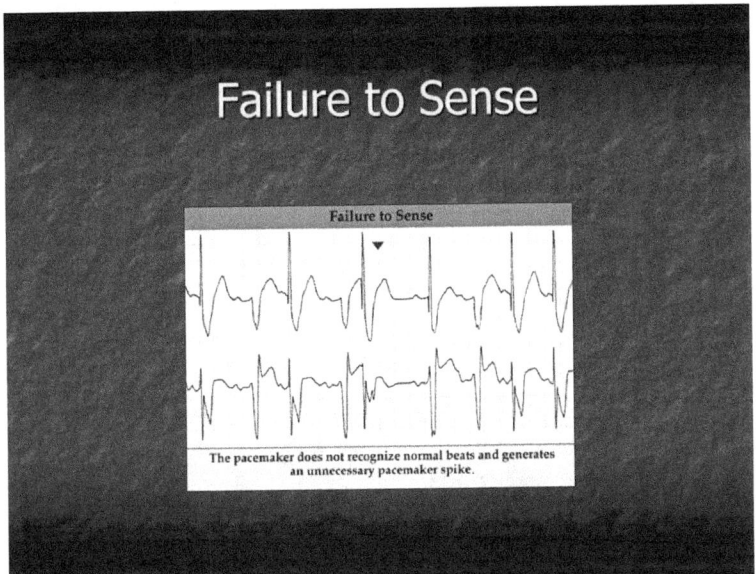

Ventricular Pacing

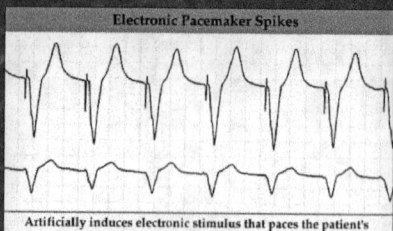

Electronic Pacemaker Spikes

Artificially induces electronic stimulus that paces the patient's rhythm causing a blip or spike on the ECG waveform

What QRS morphology is seen with an RV pacemaker?

While this tutorial is just the beginning of what one needs to know to care for patients with pacemakers, it provides the essentials to allow you to begin that journey.

www.ingramcontent.com/pod-product-compliance
Lightning Source LLC
Chambersburg PA
CBHW070847220526
45466CB00002B/911